Hemochromatosis Diet Guide

A Balanced Diet Guide To Lower Iron Consumption, Handle Symptoms, And Feel Fantastic And Living Well With Hemochromatosis

Vincenza Heaney

Table of Contents

CHAPTER ONE

Introduction

Hemochromatosis is a genetic disorder characterized by excessive absorption and storage of iron in the body. This condition causes the body to absorb too much iron from the food you eat, leading to a buildup of iron in various organs, particularly the liver, heart, pancreas, and joints.

This happens because the body absorbs more iron than it needs from the food you eat and then stores it in various organs, such as the liver, pancreas, heart, and joints.

There are different types of hemochromatosis, but the most common form is hereditary hemochromatosis (HH), which is caused by mutations in certain genes that control how much iron the body absorbs from food. The most well-known gene associated with hereditary hemochromatosis is the HFE gene.

This condition leads to an overload of iron in the body, which can cause various health issues:

Organ Damage: Excess iron can damage organs, particularly the liver, heart, pancreas, and joints. It can lead to conditions like cirrhosis (liver damage), diabetes (due to pancreatic damage), heart problems, and joint pain.

Skin Discoloration: In some cases, the skin may develop a bronze or grayish color due to excess iron deposition.

Symptoms and Effects

Early Symptoms: Initially, symptoms might not be evident. Over time, they can include fatigue, joint pain, and abdominal pain.

Organ Damage: Excess iron can lead to damage in the liver (cirrhosis), pancreas (diabetes), heart (arrhythmias, cardiomyopathy), and other organs.

Skin Discoloration: In some cases, the skin may take on a bronze or gray color.

Diagnosis and Treatment

Diagnosis: Blood tests measuring serum ferritin levels and transferrin saturation are commonly used to diagnose hemochromatosis.

Treatment: Treatment typically involves regular removal of blood (phlebotomy) to reduce iron levels. Diet changes, such as avoiding iron supplements and foods high in iron, may also be recommended.

Management

Managing hemochromatosis involves:

Regular Monitoring: Continuous monitoring of iron levels and organ function is essential.

Genetic Counseling: Understanding your genetic predisposition and family history is crucial.

Diagnosis of hemochromatosis involves blood tests to measure the levels of iron in the blood, particularly serum ferritin and transferrin saturation levels. Treatment often includes regular removal of blood (phlebotomy) to reduce iron levels and prevent further complications. Additionally, dietary changes, such as avoiding iron supplements and foods rich in iron, might be recommended.

Causes

Hemochromatosis primarily arises due to genetic mutations that affect the body's regulation of iron absorption. The main cause is an inherited mutation in specific genes that control how the body absorbs and stores iron. The most commonly associated genes are HFE, HJV, HAMP, and TFR2.

There are two primary types of hemochromatosis:

Hereditary Hemochromatosis (HH): This is the most common form and is usually caused by a mutation in the HFE gene. It's inherited in an autosomal recessive pattern, meaning both parents must pass on a defective gene for a child to develop the condition.

Secondary Hemochromatosis: This form is usually the result of other conditions such as thalassemia, chronic liver disease, or frequent blood transfusions.

Risk Factors

Genetics: The primary risk factor is having certain genetic mutations associated with hemochromatosis. This condition is more common in people of

Northern European descent, particularly those of Celtic heritage.

Family History: Having a close relative with hemochromatosis increases the risk of inheriting the mutated gene.

Gender: Men are more likely than women to develop iron overload, as women naturally lose iron through menstruation and childbirth.

Age: Symptoms of hemochromatosis might not appear until middle age or later, although iron accumulation begins earlier.

Symptoms

Early Symptoms: The symptoms of hemochromatosis can vary and might not appear until later stages when iron levels in the body have significantly increased. They can include:

Fatigue: Feeling constantly tired and lacking energy.

Joint Pain: Especially in the hands.

Abdominal Pain: Discomfort or pain in the upper right area of the abdomen.

Loss of Libido: Decreased interest in sex.

Later-Stage Symptoms:

Liver Issues: Such as cirrhosis, which can lead to symptoms like jaundice, fluid buildup in the abdomen (ascites), and liver enlargement?

Heart Problems: Including irregular heartbeat (arrhythmias) and cardiomyopathy.

Diabetes: Due to damage to the pancreas.

Skin Changes: Bronze or grayish coloration.

CHAPTER TWO

Diagnosis

Blood Tests: Measurement of serum ferritin and transferrin saturation levels to check for elevated iron levels in the blood.

Genetic Testing: To identify mutations in genes associated with hereditary hemochromatosis.

Liver Biopsy: In some cases, a biopsy might be recommended to assess the extent of liver damage.

Treatment Approaches

Treatment for hemochromatosis primarily aims to reduce the excess iron levels in the body and manage associated complications. Here are the main approaches:

Therapeutic Phlebotomy:

Therapeutic phlebotomy is the primary treatment for reducing excess iron levels in individuals with hemochromatosis. This procedure involves the removal of blood from the body, akin to blood donation, with the specific aim of reducing the iron overload.

Iron Chelation Therapy:

Iron chelation therapy is an alternative treatment for managing iron overload in individuals with conditions like hemochromatosis, particularly when therapeutic phlebotomy is not feasible or sufficient. This therapy involves the use of medications that bind to excess iron in the body, forming a complex that can be eliminated through urine or stool.

Types of Iron Chelators:

Deferoxamine: Often administered through infusion or injection, it's effective but requires frequent administration.

Deferiprone: Taken orally, it's an alternative to deferoxamine and can be more convenient for some individuals.

Deferasirox: Another oral option, taken as a tablet or suspension, providing a convenient alternative to infusion-based therapies.

Use Cases:

When Phlebotomy Isn't Possible: In cases where frequent phlebotomy isn't feasible due to health conditions or other limitations, chelation therapy might be considered.

Combination Therapy: Sometimes, a combination of therapeutic phlebotomy and iron chelation therapy might be used, especially in cases where iron levels are extremely high.

Managing Complications

Managing complications associated with hemochromatosis involves addressing specific issues that might arise due to excessive iron accumulation in various organs. Here's how complications can be managed:

Liver Complications:

Liver Cirrhosis: Treatment focuses on managing symptoms and preventing further liver damage. This might involve medications, lifestyle changes (such as limiting alcohol consumption), and monitoring for potential complications like liver cancer.

Heart Complications:

Arrhythmias and Cardiomyopathy: Treatment might involve medications to manage heart rhythm and function.

Lifestyle changes, such as a heart-healthy diet and exercise, are also crucial.

Diabetes Management:

Pancreatic Damage: If diabetes develops, appropriate management through diet, exercise, medications, and insulin therapy might be necessary.

Joint Pain:

Pain Management: Medications or physical therapy might be recommended to manage joint pain associated with hemochromatosis.

Regular Monitoring:

Health Check-ups: Regular visits to healthcare professionals for monitoring iron levels, organ function, and overall health are crucial to catch and address complications early.

Specialist Consultation:

Specialist Involvement: Depending on the complications, involvement of specialists such as hepatologists (liver specialists), cardiologists, endocrinologists, or rheumatologists might be necessary for comprehensive management.

Lifestyle Changes:

Diet and Exercise: Following a balanced diet, limiting alcohol intake, and engaging in regular exercise can help manage complications and improve overall health.

Genetic Counseling:

Family Planning: For individuals with hereditary hemochromatosis, genetic counseling helps in understanding the genetic implications for family planning and identifying at-risk relatives.

Managing complications associated with hemochromatosis often requires a multidisciplinary approach involving healthcare professionals from various specialties. Treatment and management plans are tailored to each individual's specific complications, overall health, and response to treatment. Regular monitoring and proactive management can significantly improve outcomes and quality of life for individuals with hemochromatosis.

CHAPTER THREE

Organ Damage and Implications

Hemochromatosis, particularly when left untreated or unmanaged, can lead to organ damage due to the excessive accumulation of iron. The primary organs affected by iron overload include the liver, heart, pancreas, and joints.

Liver Damage:

Cirrhosis: Excess iron in the liver can lead to cirrhosis, which is characterized by scarring and poor liver function. This can eventually lead to liver failure if not managed.

Heart Complications:

Cardiomyopathy: Iron overload can cause damage to the heart muscle, leading to cardiomyopathy, a condition where the heart becomes weak and unable to pump blood effectively.

Arrhythmias: Abnormal heart rhythms might develop due to iron deposition in the heart tissues.

Pancreatic Damage:

Diabetes: Damage to the pancreas can lead to diabetes, as the organ might struggle to produce insulin effectively.

Joint Problems:

Arthritis: Iron deposition in the joints can lead to joint pain and arthritis-like symptoms.

Implications:

Compromised Organ Function: Organ damage can lead to decreased functionality, impacting overall health and potentially leading to organ failure.

Increased Risk of Cancer: Long-standing liver damage might increase the risk of liver cancer.

Management:

Treatment Focus: Managing hemochromatosis primarily involves reducing iron levels to prevent further organ damage and managing complications as they arise.

Regular Monitoring: Continuous monitoring of organ function and iron levels is crucial for early detection and management of complications.

Lifestyle Changes: Diet modifications, exercise, and limiting alcohol consumption can help manage and prevent further complications.

Prevention:

Early Diagnosis and Treatment: Detecting and managing hemochromatosis early can significantly reduce the risk of severe organ damage.

Genetic Counseling: Understanding genetic predisposition and family history can guide prevention strategies and early intervention.

Cardiac Issues and Hemochromatosis

Hemochromatosis can lead to various cardiac issues due to the accumulation of excess iron in the heart tissues. These issues primarily include:

Cardiomyopathy:

Cardiomyopathy is a condition where the heart muscle becomes weakened or enlarged, impacting its ability to pump blood effectively.

Iron Overload Impact: Excess iron deposition in the heart can damage the muscle cells, leading to cardiomyopathy.

Symptoms: Shortness of breath, fatigue, swelling in the legs or abdomen, and irregular heartbeats (arrhythmias) might occur.

Arrhythmias:

Irregular Heart Rhythms: Iron overload can disrupt the normal electrical signals in the heart, leading to arrhythmias.

Types: These irregular heart rhythms might manifest as palpitations, rapid heartbeat, or a fluttering sensation in the chest.

Heart Failure:

Impact of Iron Accumulation: Over time, iron deposition in the heart can lead to heart failure, where the heart is unable to pump blood efficiently to meet the body's needs.

Diagnosis and Management:

Monitoring: Regular cardiac monitoring through electrocardiograms (ECGs) and echocardiograms can detect abnormalities in heart rhythm and function.

Treatment: Management involves addressing the underlying cause by reducing iron levels through therapies like phlebotomy or iron chelation. Medications might also be prescribed to manage symptoms or heart function.

Lifestyle Changes:

Diet and Exercise: A heart-healthy diet and regular exercise can support overall heart health and help manage symptoms.

Specialist Involvement:

Cardiologist Consultation: Individuals with hemochromatosis might benefit from regular consultations with cardiologists to monitor cardiac health and address any emerging issues promptly.

Prevention:

Early Intervention: Early diagnosis and management of hemochromatosis are crucial in preventing severe cardiac complications. Regular screening and monitoring for cardiac issues are recommended for individuals with hemochromatosis.

CHAPTER FOUR

Joint Pain and Arthritis

Joint pain and arthritis are potential complications of hemochromatosis due to the deposition of excess iron in the joints, leading to inflammation and damage.

Joint pain and arthritis associated with hemochromatosis can vary in severity among individuals. Effective management involves reducing iron levels, addressing joint symptoms, and collaborating with healthcare professionals, especially rheumatologists when joint issues become a concern. Early intervention and close monitoring can help mitigate the impact of joint-related complications in individuals with hemochromatosis.

Lifestyle Modifications

Lifestyle modifications can significantly support the management of hemochromatosis, particularly in controlling iron levels and reducing the risk of complications. Here are key lifestyle changes that can help:

Diet Modifications:

Limit Iron-Rich Foods: Reduce intake of red meat, organ meats, iron-fortified foods, and supplements high in iron.

Balanced Diet: Focus on a well-rounded diet with plenty of fruits, vegetables, whole grains, and lean proteins.

Calcium and Coffee/Tea: Consuming calcium-rich foods separately from iron-rich meals can inhibit iron absorption. Consuming tea or coffee separately from meals can also limit iron absorption.

Alcohol Moderation:

Limit Alcohol Consumption: Excessive alcohol can exacerbate liver damage associated with hemochromatosis. Moderate alcohol intake is advisable.

Hydration:

Stay Hydrated: Maintain adequate hydration, especially before and after therapeutic phlebotomy sessions to prevent dizziness or lightheadedness.

Avoid Supplements Without Consultation:

Iron Supplements: Avoid iron supplements unless specifically recommended by a healthcare professional.

Regular Exercise:

Physical Activity: Engage in regular, moderate exercise to support overall health. Consult with a healthcare provider to determine appropriate exercise routines.

Monitoring and Compliance:

Regular Check-ups: Attend regular medical check-ups to monitor iron levels, organ function, and overall health.

Adherence to Treatment: Comply with prescribed treatment plans, including therapeutic phlebotomy or iron chelation therapy, as advised by healthcare professionals.

Avoid Smoking:

Smoking Cessation: If applicable, quitting smoking can positively impact overall health, especially for individuals with hemochromatosis.

Genetic Counseling and Family Planning:

Family Discussions: Consider discussing genetic implications with family members for family planning decisions.

Dietary Guidelines for Hemochromatosis

Dietary adjustments can help manage iron levels in individuals with hemochromatosis. Here are some dietary guidelines:

Foods to Limit or Avoid:

Red Meat: Minimize consumption of beef, lamb, and pork, which are high in heme iron.

Organ Meats: Avoid or limit intake of liver, kidneys, and other organ meats, as they are exceptionally high in iron.

Iron-Fortified Foods: Reduce consumption of fortified cereals, bread, and processed foods containing added iron.

Moderation:

Shellfish: Consume shellfish like shrimp, clams, and mussels in moderation due to their iron content.

Iron Supplements: Avoid iron supplements unless specifically prescribed by a healthcare professional.

Iron Absorption Inhibitors:

Calcium-Rich Foods: Consume calcium-rich foods separately from iron-rich meals to inhibit iron absorption.

Tea and Coffee: Consuming these beverages separately from meals can limit iron absorption due to compounds that hinder absorption.

Balanced Diet Approach:

Fruits and Vegetables: Incorporate a variety of fruits and vegetables into your diet for essential nutrients and antioxidants.

Whole Grains: Opt for whole grains such as brown rice, quinoa, and whole wheat products.

Lean Proteins: Choose lean sources of protein like poultry, fish, and plant-based protein sources.

Cooking Methods:

Avoid Cast-Iron Cookware: Limit using cast-iron cookware for cooking, as it can increase the iron content of food.

Hydration:

Stay Hydrated: Maintain adequate hydration, as it supports overall health and well-being.

Exercise and Wellness

Exercise and overall wellness practices are beneficial for individuals managing hemochromatosis. Here's how they can contribute to better health:

Benefits of Exercise:

Improved Cardiovascular Health: Regular exercise can enhance heart health, which is crucial for individuals with hemochromatosis, as they might be at risk for heart complications.

Weight Management: Maintaining a healthy weight through exercise helps prevent obesity-related issues, which can exacerbate certain complications.

Joint Health: Low-impact exercises can support joint health and flexibility, potentially alleviating joint pain associated with hemochromatosis.

Exercise Recommendations:

Moderate Exercise: Engage in moderate-intensity exercises like brisk walking, cycling, swimming, or low-impact aerobics.

Strength Training: Include strength training exercises using light weights or resistance bands to build muscle strength.

Flexibility Exercises: Incorporate stretching exercises to improve flexibility and reduce joint stiffness.

Wellness Practices:

Stress Management: Practices like meditation, yoga, or deep breathing exercises can help manage stress, which is beneficial for overall well-being.

Adequate Sleep: Ensure sufficient and quality sleep as it supports the body's healing and overall health.

Hydration: Maintain proper hydration levels for optimal bodily function and health.

Conclusion

Managing hemochromatosis requires a multi-faceted approach, involving medical interventions, dietary adjustments, regular monitoring, genetic understanding, lifestyle modifications, and support from healthcare professionals. Adherence to treatment plans, along with a balanced lifestyle, significantly contributes to effective management, reducing the risk of complications and promoting overall

well-being.

THE END

www.ingramcontent.com/pod-product-compliance
Lightning Source LLC
Chambersburg PA
CBHW061313250726
48653CB00002B/919